CANCER, MEET THE CURE!

Michelle Cole

Write World Publishing Group
3839 McKinney Avenue
Suite: 155-373
Dallas, TX 75204

Writeworld@cs.com

Author Contact: info@MichelleCole.org

Never Bring Fear to A Cancer Fight! (Cancer Support Group):
https://www.facebook.com/groups/160987074854/

ISBN: 978-0-9722173-4-7

Write World
"we write the books that make the whole world read!"®

Books by Michelle Cole:

LILLA BELLE THE FIRST STAGES

F.A.T. CHANCE

COVID-19

VENGEANCE (**Upcoming Thriller)

*****

This book is dedicated to the strongest person that I have ever known, **my beautiful** mother, *Lillie Mae Cole, **"Mommie."**

THE FAITH EQUATION

Let's start with a little math …

"Prayer, minus worry, equals faith in God."

~Michelle Cole

Money can buy the best doctors and the best medicine, but it can't buy good health. Nor can it buy life. There is only One who can give life and good health. He is the Greatest Physician of all, the Great I Am! **God can do what doctors and medical science cannot do.** There is nothing that happens in our lives that is out of God's control. Nor does *anything* take Him by surprise.

✳✳✳✳✳

Doctor: "There is nothing more that we can do."

God: "I Am the Lord, God of all flesh. Is there anything too hard for Me?" (Jeremiah 32:27)

"And the Lord God formed man from the dust of the ground, and breathed into his nostrils the breath of life: and man became a living soul" (Genesis 2:7). Just as God gave life in the beginning, He is *still* the Giver of Life. God, alone, has the power to create life and take life.

God is the Source of <u>all</u> healing.

We seem to have forgotten that God is the Creator and Lord over all things, including life and death. We seem to have also forgotten God. Great technology and medical science will never replace God. Man is not greater than His Maker.

There is not a disease, today, that God didn't already know about. He is an all-seeing God. Nothing is hidden from Him. He knows *every* detail of the past, present and future.

Man will never be ahead of God.

"I am Alpha and Omega, the beginning and the end," saith the Lord, "which is, which was, and which is to come, the Almighty" (Revelation 1:8).

"We are God-made, not self-made."

The One who made the body can surely heal the body.

"In whose hand *is* the soul of every living thing, and the breath of all mankind" (Job 12:10).

"The Spirit of God has made me, and the breath of the Almighty gives me life" (Job 33:4).

God is not just our Creator. He is also the Giver and Sustainer – of life.

*****

LORD OVER LIFE AND DEATH

"Now see that I, even I, Am He, And there is no God besides Me. I kill and I make alive; I wound and I heal; Nor is there any who can deliver from My hand" (Deuteronomy 32:39).

God's Word will never be outdated or superceded. "Heaven and earth will pass away, but My words will never pass away" (Matthew 24:35).

The best medicine is God's Word. God's Word is *the* best prescription for all things life. There isn't a problem that we face today, or will ever face, that God does not address in His Word. God's Word is full of power, life and wisdom.

If you are seeing a doctor and getting chemotherapy and radiation treatments, there is absolutely nothing wrong with that. However, always pray, read the Bible and stay focused on the Doctor of All Doctors – Jehovah Rapha (God.) The Healer and Giver of Life. Focus on God, not your cancer.

God's power is limitless. Natural medicine has its limits.

God's Word is medicine to all flesh. However, many of us have transferred our faith, from God, to the medical profession. Use of medical science, should not interfere with faith, or our desire for God to heal us.

Instead of being prideful, we should thank God for all things, including medical advances. After all, He created the human mind. He also created the brain. We cannot do anything – without Him.

✶✶✶✶✶

"How long am I going to live?" Millions of people are diagnosed with cancer. There are many types of this life-threatening disease. For those with cancer, fear spreads like wildfire. The fear of death immediately surfaces. I certainly understand what it's like. I have been there. However, instead of thinking about writing your will, **have the will to live!** The will to fight! Don't allow fear to paralyze you. Fear can actually do more harm than the cancer itself. Replace your fear – with faith.

*****

In October of 1997, an X-ray revealed a tumor near my heart and my left lung. At the time, I was 27 years old. My family was worried. They were also scared. Worry and fear often go hand-in-hand. I remained calm. Many could not understand why. Why was I so calm?

MY DISCOVERY

As I was leaving work one morning, a pickup truck was backing up towards my car. It was very obvious that the driver did not see me. Instead of honking my horn, immediately, to get the driver's attention, I sat there. Frozen. I couldn't move. The truck bumped my car. No one was hurt.

In spite of the very minor accident, I went to see a chiropractor. Minor accidents can cause problems. The chiropractor took X-rays of my spine and chest.

Before I left the chiropractor's office, he explained my X-ray results to me. My chest X-ray was abnormal. He told me there was a large mass present in my chest, on the left side; near my heart and my left lung. "Possibly pneumonia." He recommended that I see my primary care physician as soon as possible.

Shortly after leaving the chiropractor's office, I called and scheduled an appointment with my primary care physician. I was able to see him the next day.

*****

A CT scan of my chest was taken the following day. Pneumonia was ruled out. I was told that the mass was either benign (noncancerous) or malignant (cancerous). I was certainly praying that it was benign. My doctor scheduled a biopsy. The biopsy would reveal if the mass was benign or malignant. If the mass was cancerous, the doctors could also determine the type and the grade (how aggressive my cancer was).

*****

My first biopsy was a needle-biopsy. The same-day procedure was very short; about 30 minutes. Unfortunately, it did not provide the answers that the doctors and I were needing.

I had to undergo a second biopsy. This biopsy would be incisional. I still have the scar, to this day. Although a scar is cosmetic, it is still an awesome reminder of what God did for me! I thank God for doing what only He could do – heal me.

God does not panic. Why should we?

I was hospitalized on a Friday. The incisional biopsy took place later that afternoon. I was kept in the hospital overnight. The second biopsy was successful. It provided the information that the doctors and I needed.

*****

The next morning, a doctor came into my hospital room and gave my parents and me the dreaded news. The mass was malignant. I had cancer. Non-Hodgkin lymphoma (also known as non-Hodgkin's lymphoma or NHL). It's a cancer that starts in white blood cells called lymphocytes. Lymphocytes are a part of the body's immune system. The doctor also told us what the next steps were.

When the doctor left, my father went to the bathroom, in my hospital room, and cried. It wasn't the news that we were praying and hoping for. I remained calm. I was also ready to go home. I was released from the hospital later that morning.

*****

Was I going to die? Reality is, we are all going to die. One day. You don't have to be ill. You can be healthy and young and still die. There are many people who die, every day, who don't have cancer or a life-threatening illness. Death can be around the corner for any of us.

Why was I so calm? I knew that God was my life support. And He still is. I knew that God made my body, therefore, I knew that He could easily fix it. *Anything*, that was wrong with it. I knew that He could heal me. And I hoped and prayed that He would.

*****

I underwent 6 months of chemotherapy treatments followed by 6 weeks of radiation treatments. I lost all of my hair, but I **never lost my faith in God.** Nor did I ever lose hope. Faith in God can work wonders! It is what brought me through one of the biggest storms of my life. Without faith in God, I would have fallen apart. I would have been a basket case.

I didn't live like I was going to die. I lived like I was going to live. And if you have cancer, it is very important that you do the same.

Yes, I had **cancer**, but it **did not have me.** God had me. And He also has you.

Life is full of unknowns. Only God knows what the outcome will be. He has the last say. **All things are in His hands.** Not ours. Not the doctors'. Only His. Knowing this can make a huge difference, when we face any storm in life. And there are many. It is 14 years later. **I thank God for sparing my life!**

"I Am the Lord that healeth thee" (Exodus 15:26).

*****

AFTER HEARING THE NEWS

Please don't allow anyone to tell you how to grieve, or how to behave when hearing, "you have cancer." Everyone is different. If you want to cry, go ahead and cry. If you are scared, admit it. Angry? That's fine, also. Being honest is crucial. Do what works best for you, as long as it's not anything that is harmful. Hearing the news can be devastating. What you do, **after hearing the news,** is very important. *What now?*

THE MIND

The mind is very powerful. It is captain of the body. It is crucial to have a positive mindset. Have a, "I'm *going* to survive," mentality. Surround yourself with positive people. Do not surround yourself with negative people.

Your doctor should also have a positive mindset. If you are not comfortable or happy with your doctor, replace him or her. Because it really *is* – all about you. Your health. Your well-being.

SUPPORT

Support is much-needed. Oftentimes, those joining you in your fight are: your spouse or significant other, family members, friends, your medical team and cancer support groups ... However, the first human being joining in your fight against cancer is – **YOU.** You **are your most important advocate.** If anyone noticed that I did not mention **God,** relax; He *is* already **there.** He never leaves us. Nor will He ever forsake us. For those of you who have little, or no support, always remember ... If all you have is God, you have more than enough!

LIFE AND DEATH

For some of us, when we think that death may be close, it is only then that life becomes important. Death can be close for any of us, without being diagnosed with cancer. However, sometimes, it is not until something threatens our life, or we have a near-death experience, that we seem to realize what a blessing life truly is! God breathes life into every human being. We are all on His ventilator. **God is our Supreme life support.**

"YOU HAVE CANCER"

Two questions often come to mind when being told those 3 dreaded words – you have cancer:

"Am I going to die?"

"How long am I going to live?"

Almost immediately, we are paralyzed with fear. Hearing the words, "you have cancer," is like a death sentence. It is devastating news. However, it is very important to do **2 things:**

> ➢ **Focus on God's Word, not your doctor's report.**
> ➢ **Replace fear with FAITH!**

We have faith in doctors, airline pilots, bus drivers ... Why is it that we have so *little* faith – in the All-Powerful God?

Our faith cannot be in anything, or anyone, our **faith** must be **in God.** He is the One who gives life to every human being. He is also the Sustainer of Life. A cancer diagnosis may have surprised you, however, it did not surprise God. He is never taken by surprise. There is nothing that He doesn't see. There is nothing that He doesn't know. And there is, nothing, that He cannot do! God is all-powerful, He is all-knowing and He is in control – of all things!

God created our bodies, therefore, He can fix anything that is wrong. If you have a BMW and it breaks down, you wouldn't take it to a Ford dealership because they didn't make the vehicle, nor are their technicians trained to work on bimmers. You would take your BMW to a BMW dealership.

*****

God didn't just create man. He created the world and everything that dwells in it. He also governs the world, therefore, cancer is not a problem for Him!

"God doesn't need a Plan B. He *never* fails!"

FEAR OR FAITH?

It is very important to replace your fear – with faith. You can't have both at the same time. There is only room for one. You must choose one or the other. I hope that you **choose – FAITH.**

- ➤ **Faith focuses on God.** Fear focuses on cancer.
- ➤ **Faith focuses on God's Word.** Fear focuses on the doctor's report.
- ➤ **Faith empowers!** Fear cowers.
- ➤ **Faith looks** up (**to God**). Fear drags you down.
- ➤ **Faith screams, "yes, I can!"** Fear screams, "no, you can't!"
- ➤ **Faith gives** you a **peace** of mind. Fear clouds the mind with worry.

"In the midst of any storm, be not dismayed; the Son is there!"

PETER

Many of us are like Peter. As long as we are focused on Jesus, the Great I Am, we are at peace and doing just fine. The moment that we take our eyes off of, Jesus, fear sets in and we begin to sink. The lesson learned from that story is simple – **keep your eyes on, Jesus, don't focus on the** cancer **storm.** The wind and the waves obey His will. Why do some think that cancer is bigger than God? There is nothing too big for Almighty God. When we focus on the cancer, that is exactly what we are saying.

God rewards faith.

Storms are a part of life. For each of us. How you respond to storms is crucial. Don't cower in fear. Stand strong in faith, knowing that Jesus is your Anchor. He can calm any storm. He can also remove any storm. He can do – anything. God knows if you have faith. If you need more faith, just ask Him; He will increase your faith!

"Faith comes by hearing, hearing by the Word of God" (Romans 10:17).

God does *not* want us to worry; He wants us to have faith in Him.

"Who of you by worrying can add a single hour to his life?" (Luke 12:25).

CHOOSING THE RIGHT ONCOLOGIST

One of the most important decisions to make is choosing the right doctor. Who is the *right* doctor?

- ➤ One who gives hope, not one who stamps out hope.
- ➤ One who treats you, the human being, first and foremost. The disease needs no hope or encouragement; the person battling cancer does.
- ➤ One who takes the time to address all of your questions and concerns.
- ➤ One who is honest with you, optimistic and keeps you well-informed.

If the doctor treats the individual; the disease will automatically be treated. *The individual and the disease are inseparable.

BE YOUR OWN ADVOCATE!

You are your best advocate. No one should be as passionate about your well-being as you are. Don't be a passive participant. Take a very active role in your cancer care. Being an advocate can help you move from being a patient to a survivor. It can give you a sense of control amidst fear and uncertainty. Focus on what you can control. Do thorough research about your cancer. Write down any questions or concerns that you have and discuss them with your doctor:

> ➤ What type of cancer do I have?
> ➤ What stage is my cancer?
> ➤ What are the best treatment options for me?
> ➤ What are the short-term effects and long-term effects?
> ➤ What are next steps?

**Always *remember*, God CANCER!

*****

WHY IS GOD THE CURE?

- ➢ **God is** omnipotent **(all-powerful)** which means that He can do anything.
- ➢ **God is** omniscient **(all-knowing).** There is *nothing* that He doesn't know. He is never taken by surprise. He sees the past, present and future – simultaneously.
- ➢ **God is** omnipresent; **(He is present everywhere).**

The words, omnipotent, omniscient and omnipresent are attributes that belong solely to Almighty God. God's timing and choices are absolutely, perfect. Trust Him!

GOD'S TIMING

God is not bound by time. In fact, He controls time. Oftentimes, doctors tell cancer patients how long they are going to live. No one knows when anyone is going to die. Only our Creator knows. Your doctor doesn't even know how long he or she will live. No amount of college, or medical degrees, will take God's place. God knows how human beings measure time. However, God is not moved by time. Time is of no concern to the All-Powerful **God**. Why? Because He **controls – everything.** Including, time.

"But beloved, be not ignorant of this one thing, that one day, is with the Lord as a thousand years, and a thousand years as one day" (2 Peter 3:8).

TOO LATE?

Remember, Lazarus? Lazarus was dead. Jesus was the Difference Maker then and He is the Difference Maker now. And always. Jesus purposely let Lazarus die so that non-believers would believe and to prove that nothing is too hard for Him. Another important **note: there is no such thing as too late with God.** He is Alpha and Omega. He is the All-Powerful God. His power is limitless. Boundless. And so is His wisdom and His knowledge.

DAVID

We will all experience Goliaths in life – problems and circumstances that are huge and very serious in nature. Goliath's size didn't frighten David. Why? Because David knew the size of his God. David didn't focus on the giant; he focused on the One who made the giant. God made David victorious. He rewarded David's faith.

MOSES

Pharoah had worldly-power and armies of men. Moses had the One who made the world and everything that dwells in it. **If God is on your side, you will *never* lose.** What awesome miracles God performed, including one of my favorites – parting the Red Sea. God easily parted the Red Sea, because after all, He created that sea. No one or nothing is any match for God. His power is unmatched. When we are in God's hands, we are in the very Best of Hands!

JOB

"Though He slay me, yet will I trust Him: but I will maintain my own ways before Him" (Job 13:15).

Job went through enormous pain and suffering. Unimaginable pain and suffering. And even though Job didn't understand why all of the horrible things were happening to him, he kept his faith in God. Job knew that God controls all things. And He still does. God did not allow Satan to take Job's life. Another example that **God is in control, of all things, including life and death.** God gave Job twice as much as he had before. God restored his health and blessed him with a very long life – after all of his pain and suffering.

*****

We will not always have the same ending, but God requires the same thing from each of us – have faith in Him. Sovereign God knows what is best and He will do what is best.

Some of you may be saying, "Michelle, that was then, and this is now. That was eons ago. Times have changed." Times may change, however, God *never* does. "Jesus Christ is the same yesterday, today and forevermore" (Hebrews 13:8).

Only God knows how things are going to turn out. However, have faith and remember …

**God <u>has</u> the final say. Trust Him!

✳✳✳✳✳

SCRIPTURES ON GOD'S SOVEREIGNTY

"For nothing will be impossible with God." (Luke 1:37)

"For by Him all things were created, in heaven and on earth, visible and invisible, whether thrones or dominions or rulers or authorities — all things were created through Him and for Him. And He is before all things, and in Him all things hold together." (Colossians 1:16–17)

"Whatever the Lord pleases, He does, In heaven and in earth, in the seas and in all deeps." (Psalm 135:6)

"See now that I, even I, am He, and there is no god besides Me. I kill, and I make alive; I wound, and I heal; neither is there any that can deliver out of My hand." (Deuteronomy 32:39)

"Fixing our eyes on Jesus, The Author and Perfecter of Faith, who for the joy set before Him endured the cross, despising the shame, and has sat down at the right hand of the throne of God." (Hebrews 12:2)

"Even from eternity, I am He, and there is none who can deliver out of My hand; I act and who can reverse it?" (Isaiah 43:13)

"I know that You can do all things, and that no purpose of Yours can be thwarted." (Job 42:2)

And looking at them Jesus said to them, "With people this is impossible, but with God all things are possible." (Matthew 19:26)

"The Lord has established His throne in the heavens, and His kingdom rules over all." (Psalm 104:19)

"Heaven is My throne. And Earth is the footstool of My feet; what kind of house will you build for Me?" says the Lord. "Or what is there for My repose?" (Isaiah 66:1)

"Many are the plans in the mind of a man, but it is the purpose of the Lord that will stand." (Proverbs 19:21)

SCRIPTURES ON FEAR

"We should never fear tomorrow; Almighty God is already there." ~ *Michelle Cole*

"When I am afraid, I put my trust in You." ~ Psalm 56:3

"I prayed to the Lord, and He answered me. He freed me from all my fears." ~ Psalm 34:4

"The Lord is my light and my salvation — whom shall I fear? The Lord is the stronghold of my life — of whom shall I be afraid?" ~ Psalm 27:1

"So do not fear, for I am with you; do not be dismayed, for I am your God. I will strengthen you and help you; I will uphold you with My righteous right hand." ~ Isaiah 41:10

"For God has not given us a spirit of fear, but of power and of love and of a sound mind." ~ 2 Timothy 1:7

"Peace is what I leave with you; it is My own peace that I give you. I do not give it as the world does. Do not be worried and upset; do not be afraid." ~ John 14:27

"When anxiety was great within me, Your consolation brought joy to my soul." ~ Psalm 94:19

"An anxious heart weighs a man down, but a kind word cheers him up." ~ Proverbs 12:25

"Have I not commanded you? Be strong and courageous. Do not be terrified; do not be discouraged, for the Lord your God will be with you wherever you go." ~ Joshua 1:9

"God is our refuge and strength, an ever-present help in trouble." ~ Psalm 46:1

Dear Readers:

I hope you enjoyed reading this book as much as I enjoyed writing it.

Keep the faith! **God is much bigger than cancer.

~*Michelle Cole*

www.ingramcontent.com/pod-product-compliance
Lightning Source LLC
Chambersburg PA
CBHW022136280326
41933CB00007B/715